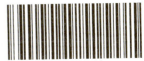

ST. FRANCIS JR. HIGH
LIBRARY
333 - 18th STREET SOUTH
LETHBRIDGE, ALBERTA
T1J 3E5

WITHDRAWN

making smart choices

making smart choices about sexual activity

Stephanie C. Perkins

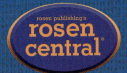

New York

*To those whose knowledge, trust, and encouragement
helped me to make my own smart choices*

Published in 2008 by The Rosen Publishing Group, Inc.
29 East 21st Street, New York, NY 10010

Copyright © 2008 by The Rosen Publishing Group, Inc.

First Edition

All rights reserved. No part of this book may be reproduced in any form without permission in writing from the publisher, except by a reviewer.

Library of Congress Cataloging-in-Publication Data

Perkins, Stephanie C.
 Making smart choices about sexual activity / Stephanie C. Perkins.—1st ed.
   p. cm.—(Making smart choices)
 Includes bibliographical references and index.
 ISBN-13: 978-1-4042-1386-9 (library binding)
 1. Sex instruction for teenagers. 2. Teenagers—Sexual behavior. I. Title.
 HQ35.P456 2008
 613.9071'2—dc22

2007029655

Manufactured in Malaysia

contents

Introduction 4

chapter one Making Choices 7

chapter two Sexual Activity and Your Options 16

chapter three Potential Consequences of Sexual Activity 26

chapter four Opportunities for Growth 36

Glossary 39

For More Information 41

For Further Reading 43

Bibliography 44

Index 47

introduction

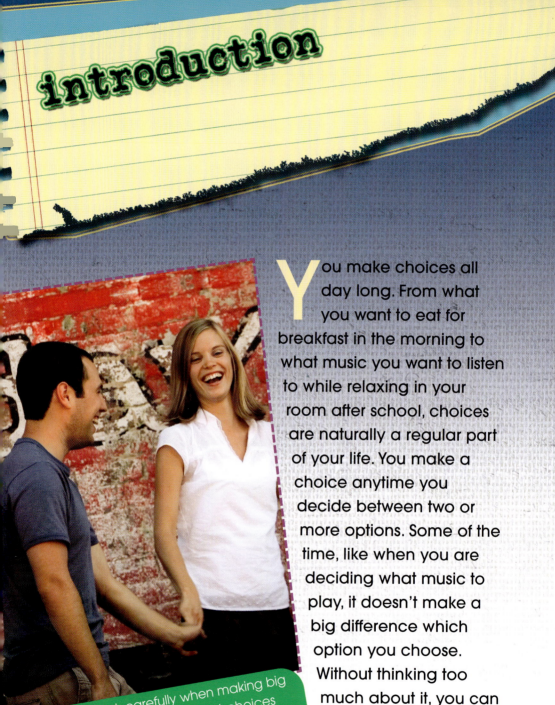

You make choices all day long. From what you want to eat for breakfast in the morning to what music you want to listen to while relaxing in your room after school, choices are naturally a regular part of your life. You make a choice anytime you decide between two or more options. Some of the time, like when you are deciding what music to play, it doesn't make a big difference which option you choose. Without thinking too much about it, you can quickly decide what you're in the mood to hear at the moment.

You must think carefully when making big decisions. You will make smart choices when you consider both the good and bad outcomes that might occur.

Introduction

If you end up not liking what you have chosen and want to hear something else, it's no big deal. You can change your mind without any negative results.

But other times, the choices you make can have a much more serious impact on your life because of the consequences that may come with them. For those more difficult choices that you have to make, it is important to weigh your options thoroughly.

Deciding whether or not you should have sex, for example, is one of those choices that is best made with a lot of consideration. Having sex requires both maturity and responsibility. If sex is not practiced safely, it can lead to undesirable consequences, such as unintended pregnancies and sexually transmitted diseases (STDs). The choice to have sex cannot be made as easily and quickly as your choice of tunes. Instead, this decision must be made by taking into consideration all the possible outcomes, both physical and emotional, that can arise from having a sexual relationship.

It is important to be thoughtful when making the big decisions in your life. Those choices help to shape your identity, which involves your own sense of self as well as the way other people see you. In effect, making good decisions in your life helps you to have more self-confidence just as much as it helps others to view you as a confident person who has a good head on his or her shoulders.

However, it is also very important to remember that no one ever makes all the right decisions all the time. You should not be afraid to make mistakes because mistakes

Making Smart Choices About Sexual Activity

are how we learn and how we grow into better people. At the same time, you can't make a rash or uninformed decision thinking that later you can just walk away and call it a mistake when things go wrong. Some decisions, once made, are not easily unmade.

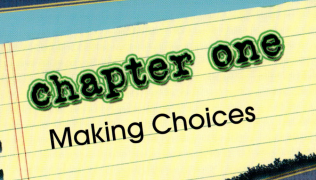

chapter one
Making Choices

Who or what influences the choices we make? There are many answers to that question, and they vary from person to person. We all have an identity or self-image, an idea of who we are and who we want to be. This self-image often drives the choices we make. But what factors shape our self-images?

The Influence of Role Models

Different factors that influence who we are include our age, sex, and ethnic background, as well as the way we were brought up and where we were brought up. But

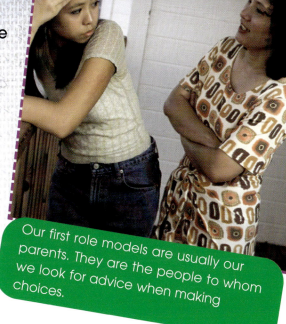

Our first role models are usually our parents. They are the people to whom we look for advice when making choices.

Making Smart Choices About Sexual Activity

perhaps the most important influences are the people in our lives who affect us directly. This group includes parents, grandparents, other family members, teachers, and mentors. It also includes our peers, such as siblings, friends, and boyfriends or girlfriends. These people who influence us are called role models. We observe how they do things, and we model our own behavior on theirs. When we come to a point at which we have to make a decision, we may even ask ourselves, "What would so-and-so do in this situation?" As with most things in life, some role models are better than others.

The Influence of the Mass Media

In addition to real-life role models, people today are greatly influenced by figures they see in the mass media. The mass media includes movies, television, music, music videos, and sports, fashion, and entertainment magazines. People in the mass media influence the way we all dress, talk, act, and view the world around us. This influence may be particularly strong when it comes to the way teens see things. For example, the media seems to be very influential when it comes to teens' views on sex and their willingness to become sexually active. According to a study published in the journal *Pediatrics*, the media often makes sex seem very glamorous to young people. You rarely see the undesirable consequences that may come with being sexually active. By doing this, the media encourages teens to believe that having sex is nothing but a good time. Unfortunately, that is not the case in the

Making Choices

real world. It doesn't make a lot of sense to rely on media figures for guidance in making personal choices.

Good Influence or Bad?

You will find that some of your influences inspire you in good ways, and others affect you in ways that aren't so good. Knowing who and what influences you in a positive way can help you to make better decisions. It's a simple equation: better decisions result in better outcomes, which result in greater happiness.

When you were younger, your parents or other adults made decisions for you. You didn't have much freedom, but neither did you have to take responsibility for any poor decisions that others made for you. In many cases now, however, making smart decisions comes down to you and nobody else. You are the one who has to live with the consequences of your decisions. So, when it comes to important decisions, such as whether or not you want to become sexually active, you can look to others for help and advice. But in the end, the decision will be yours to make. As this is the case, it's a good idea to try to understand everything you can about your options.

What Is Sexual Activity?

When someone is sexually active, it means that he or she engages in activities designed to bring sexual satisfaction. Some think of sexual activity only as sexual intercourse, or when a man inserts his penis into a woman's vagina (vaginal intercourse). But sexual activity may also include anal or oral sex. Sexual activity may also mean the touching or rubbing of the genitals, or mutual masturbation. Sex between a male and a female is heterosexual sex, while sex between two males or two females is homosexual sex.

What Is Abstinence?

When you abstain from something, you choose to avoid it. People may abstain from drinking, gambling, or anything they think will bring negative consequences. However, when used alone, the word "abstinence" usually means the avoidance of sexual intercourse. Abstinence means different things to different people. For instance, one person might decide that kissing and holding hands is OK, but engaging in any type of advanced sexual play is off-limits. Another person may be comfortable engaging in oral sex but does not want to get involved in vaginal intercourse.

Why Choose Abstinence?

There are many reasons why teens choose abstinence. Some want to wait until they are older or until marriage. Others know that they aren't yet ready to handle all the emotions and potential consequences that come with having sex. Some abstain from sex because they feel it takes energy and attention away from other matters that are more important to them, such as creative or spiritual activities, or physical training for a big event.

Some faiths forbid or strongly discourage sex before marriage, so many teens are abstinent because it fits with their religious beliefs. Teens may also be encouraged or

Making Choices

even pressured by their parents or family to refrain from (avoid) sex. Others choose abstinence because they are concerned about contracting a sexually transmitted disease (STD) or getting pregnant. All of these are good reasons to be abstinent.

Nowadays, our society is very liberated, and sexuality is not hidden like it used to be. In this atmosphere, many view abstinence as old-fashioned. The truth, however, is that abstinence never goes out of style. Choosing abstinence is a mature thing to do, and it is something anyone can do at any time, even if you have been sexually active in the past.

The Consequences of Sexual Activity

Maybe you think it's right for you to be sexually active, but you're not quite ready for vaginal intercourse. If this is the case, don't be fooled into thinking that you have made a choice that is completely safe.

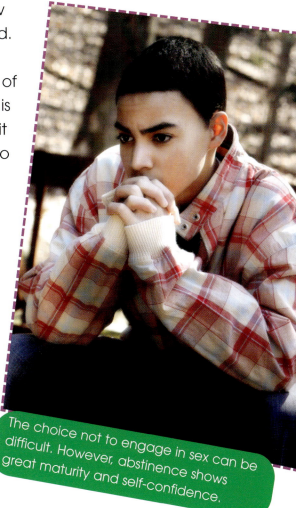

The choice not to engage in sex can be difficult. However, abstinence shows great maturity and self-confidence.

Making Smart Choices About Sexual Activity

Engaging in any form of sexual activity, including oral and anal intercourse, puts you at risk for an STD. What's worse is that many STDs have few or no outward symptoms, so it is possible that you don't even realize you have been infected. This situation can result in the STD being passed along unwittingly to another sexual partner.

If you have contracted an STD, the disease can be passed on in two ways. First, it can be spread if your genitals come in contact with your partner's genitals, anus, or mouth. Under the right circumstances, this can happen even if the skin-to-skin contact is brief. The second

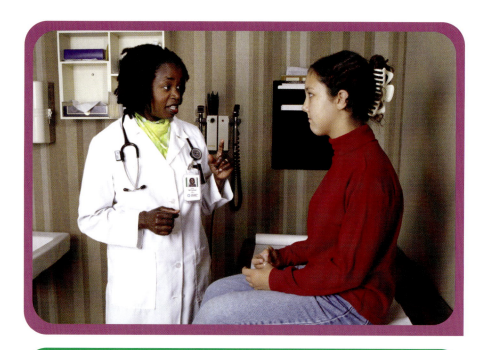

Your doctor can help you understand the health consequences of being sexually active.

Making Choices

way of transmitting an STD is through exchanging bodily fluids—including blood, vaginal fluid, pre-ejaculatory fluid, and semen.

To put it bluntly, just about every form of sexual contact carries with it the possibility of unwanted outcomes. As you may have figured out by now, there is only one level of abstinence that does not come with any unexpected consequences: total abstinence, or refraining from all sexual activity with any partner.

Different Paths

Each one of us is a unique individual. We each follow our own special path to come to the decision point, or crossroads, where we have to make a choice about our sexual activity. Here are some examples of how teens might arrive at a crossroads:

- Seventeen-year-old Marissa has always wanted to wait until she is married to have sex. But lately, her boyfriend has been pressuring her to sleep with him. Marissa loves her boyfriend, but she's afraid of having sex too soon and possibly getting pregnant or contracting an STD. Her boyfriend keeps assuring her that they will be careful, but it doesn't make her feel that much better. Even so, Marissa doesn't want to break up with her boyfriend. She has a big decision to make.
- Joel just turned fifteen. He's the first guy in his group of friends to have a serious girlfriend. Being normal

Making Smart Choices About Sexual Activity

guys, Joel and his friends are curious about sex, and so Joel's friends are constantly encouraging him to start having sex with his girlfriend. Joel is as interested in sex as his buddies, but he respects his girlfriend when she tells him that she is not ready to be intimate with him. His buddies tell him that his girlfriend will give in if he just keeps trying. In this situation, Joel must decide between wanting to honor his girlfriend's wishes and giving in to peer pressure from his friends and trying to convince his girlfriend to start having sex.

- Sixteen-year-old Angela has been dating her new boyfriend, Tony, for the past three months. Tony, who is sexually active, has promised her that he will wait until she is ready to have sex with him. However, even though Angela thinks she might be ready, she also knows that there can be unwanted consequences to having sex. Her best friend got

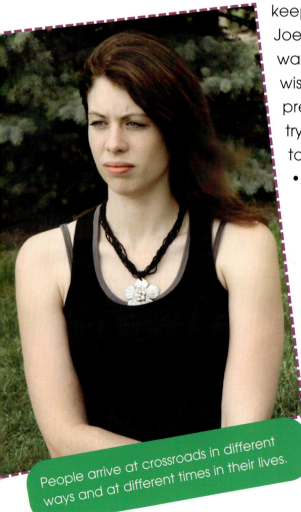

People arrive at crossroads in different ways and at different times in their lives.

14

Making Choices

pregnant last year and is now a teenage mother. Also, Angela has been talking to two of her older cousins lately. One says she waited until she was in college to start having sex, and the other says that she waited until she was married. Both of Angela's cousins say that they are glad they waited until they were older and more responsible before they became sexually active. Their stories have made Angela seriously consider remaining abstinent until she is either older or married. Still, this has put Angela at a crossroads with herself. One part of her thinks she may be ready to have sex with Tony, but another part of her isn't so sure and sees lots of good reasons to wait.

These teens followed different paths to come to the point where they had to decide if they wanted to start having sex or not. Your path may be similar to one of theirs, or it may be entirely different. Whichever path you follow to reach your own crossroads, the next step is to consider all your options and figure out which one is best for you.

chapter two
Sexual Activity and Your Options

The trend in the United States is pretty clear: teens are having less intercourse. The latest statistics from twenty-two government agencies indicate that about 45 percent of U.S. high school students (6.7 million students) reported having sexual intercourse in 2005. This is down from 54 percent in 1991. One recent study reported that about half of all American girls aged thirteen to nineteen have never had sexual intercourse.

Teen births can also be seen as an indication of sexual activity. A government report issued by the Federal

Attitudes regarding sexual activity change over time. In the United States, fewer and fewer teenage girls are opting to become mothers.

Sexual Activity and Your Options

Interagency Forum on Child and Family Statistics found that U.S. teen births were at an all-time low in 2007.

What Do I Think About Sex?

So, how do you make the decision between becoming sexually active or remaining abstinent? Making choices about big events in your life is never easy, that's for sure. Everyone has his or her own way of figuring out what is best. One good place to start is to figure out your comfort level on the subject of sex. As the wise old philosophers say, "Know thyself." Ask yourself the following questions and answer them honestly:

- When my boyfriend/girlfriend and I are kissing and he/she starts saying sexy or sexual things to me, do I start feeling uncomfortable or does it excite me?
- When my boyfriend/girlfriend touches or rubs me in a sexual way, do I want him/her to stop or slow down? Or do I enjoy it and want to go further?
- Would I be comfortable bringing up the subject of wanting to have safer sex with my boyfriend/girlfriend? Or would I be afraid to talk about it in case the guy/girl I care about might get upset?
- Am I mature enough to go to a drugstore or to a family planning clinic to obtain condoms so that my partner and I can have safer sex from the start?
- Could I bring myself to ask my boyfriend/girlfriend about his/her previous sexual activity?

Making Smart Choices About Sexual Activity

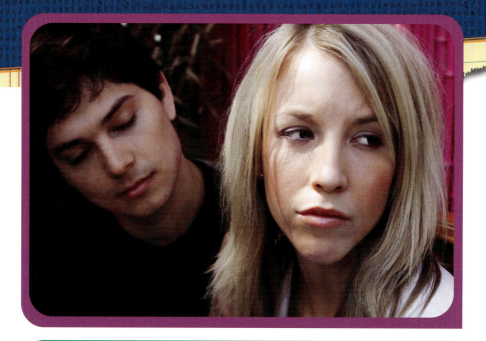

It's important to be honest with your partner as well as with yourself. If the thought of having sex makes you uncomfortable, let him or her know.

- How would I feel if I found out that I had contracted an STD? What if I contracted an STD that could not be completely cured, like herpes or HIV?
- For girls: What would I do if I got pregnant? Would the guy I'm considering having sex with step up and be responsible if he got me pregnant? Or would he probably leave me to deal with the responsibility by myself?
- For guys: What if I got my girlfriend pregnant? If she wanted to keep the baby, would I be willing to support her and our child emotionally and financially

Sexual Activity and Your Options

throughout the pregnancy and once the child is born? Would I be happy having a child and being a father while I was still in high school? Or, how would I feel if my girlfriend had an abortion without talking to me about it first?

Your answers will tell you a lot about your attitudes regarding sexual activity. Are you immediately uncomfortable thinking about the subject? You may find that you are quite comfortable talking and thinking about sexual activity and all the ways you need to be mature when deciding to have sex for the first time. Or, you may find yourself feeling uneasy when you think about everything involved in having a safe sexual relationship with another person. Both reactions are normal. The bottom line to all of this is, if you aren't comfortable when you think about the steps you need to take to be safely sexually active, then it's probably a good sign that you need more time before you choose to start having sex.

If You Choose to Become Sexually Active

Let's say you've put a lot of serious thought into the issue, and you have had an open and honest discussion about it with your boyfriend or girlfriend. Together, you have come to the decision that you are both ready to have sex. What now? How do you go about safely beginning a sexual relationship?

First, it's important to make sure that you are prepared to have safer sex when the moment finally happens. The

Making Smart Choices About Sexual Activity

importance of choosing to have safer sex cannot be stressed enough. This means that you are using one or more forms of contraceptive protection, which includes condoms, birth control pills, and spermicides. These things reduce your chances of getting pregnant or either catching or passing on a sexually transmitted disease. Using protection every time you have sex is definitely the most mature and responsible thing you can do for yourself and your partner, if you choose to become sexually active.

What Is the Best Protection?

Studies show that the latex condom is the best type of protection available. When used properly, it is up to 98 percent effective in protecting both you and your partner. Fortunately, recent government studies show that condom use is up among American teens. Of those who reported having sex during a three-month period in 2005, 63 percent (about 9 million teens) said they used a condom. This figure was only 46 percent in 1991.

Latex condoms offer dual protection, meaning they create an effective barrier against both pregnancy and STDs. Options such as birth control pills and spermicides are useful only in the prevention of pregnancy; they don't protect against STDs. For this reason, birth control pills and spermicides should be used along with a condom, not in place of one. As you know, sexually transmitted diseases are spread through bodily fluids such as blood, vaginal fluids, pre-ejaculatory fluid, and semen, or through contact

Sexual Activity and Your Options

with infected skin, in the case of skin diseases. The latex condom creates a barrier that makes it nearly impossible for STDs to get through.

In addition to latex, condoms are also made of lambskin and polyurethane. (These are mainly for people who are allergic to latex.) However, neither of these types of condoms is as effective as the latex condom in offering dual protection.

Birth Control Pills

Sometimes called "the pill," birth control pills are synthetic (manufactured) hormones that prevent a girl or woman from ovulating. Ovulation occurs when a female's ovaries release a mature egg. If an egg is fertilized by one of the millions of sperm that are produced when a man ejaculates, a pregnancy can result. When taken properly, the pill is more than 99 percent effective in preventing pregnancy. Taken improperly, however, the pill is much less effective.

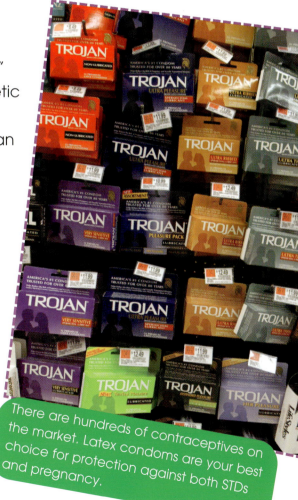

There are hundreds of contraceptives on the market. Latex condoms are your best choice for protection against both STDs and pregnancy.

Spermicides

Like condoms, spermicides are widely available at drugstores. They come in creams, gels, film, foam, and vaginal suppositories. There are also condoms that contain spermicide. All of these forms are designed to prevent pregnancy by killing the sperm that are produced when a man ejaculates.

Spermicides are effective only 50 to 94 percent of the time when used alone, and they do not provide any significant protection against STDs. For this reason, a latex condom should always be used along with a spermicide.

When Can a Woman Get Pregnant?

You may have heard that a woman can get pregnant only if she has unprotected sex during the two to three days that she is ovulating. But what you may not know is that sperm can live inside a woman's fallopian tubes and remain viable (capable of causing pregnancy) for up to six days. In addition, the egg is viable for twenty-four to forty-eight hours after ovulation. This means that, under the right circumstances, there are as many as eight days during the menstrual cycle on which a girl can get pregnant. Throw in the fact that a girl's cycle can change from month to month, and it's clear that there are no truly "safe" days to have unprotected sex. Always choose to use latex condoms and one or more other kinds of contraception every time you have sex.

Sexual Activity and Your Options

If You Choose Abstinence

Abstinence is not always an easy path to go down. You may face pressure from your friends to become sexually active. You may also have your boyfriend or your girlfriend trying to convince you to have sex before you are ready. You also may be dealing with increased sexual feelings of your own, as your sex glands become more active and release hormones. It's especially difficult if you are dealing with all of these situations!

    Choosing abstinence may improve your self-esteem, or sense of self-worth. It means that you are in touch with your feelings and that you are able to stick with what you believe is the right thing to do. There may be times when you wish you weren't abstinent, such as when you start dating someone new or when your friends might be bragging about sex. But over time, your dedication to yourself can become a source of pride. In addition, if you are waiting until you are married, you can think of your virginity as a prized gift. Giving it to your new spouse can help to create an even more special bond.

    You may decide to practice complete abstinence, meaning that you are not participating in any kind of sexual activity whatsoever. In this case, you have the added peace of mind that comes with knowing that you will not contract any sexually transmitted diseases. You have enough things to deal with when you're a teen— trying to get through school, part-time jobs, sports, and

Making Smart Choices About Sexual Activity

other extracurricular activities. So, having one less stressful thought on your mind can only make your life better.

Making Abstinence Easier

Some teens find being abstinent easier than others, and this is very normal and understandable. But there are things you can do to help keep your resolve strong. Standing firm behind a hard decision is sometimes easier if you aren't going through it alone.

You can confide in your friends who also haven't had sex yet. Even if most of your friends have become sexually

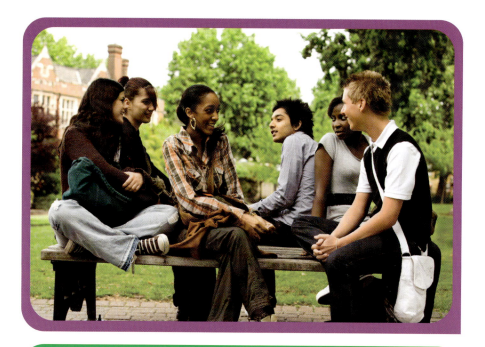

Real friends will support you in your choices. Talking with those you trust can help you to feel good about a difficult decision.

Sexual Activity and Your Options

active, chances are that you are not the only one who has not. They, too, might just be looking for someone to talk to.

You can find and join groups that support abstinence. Most are through churches or Christian-based organizations such as the Abstinence Clearinghouse. These groups support those who choose abstinence.

You can sign an abstinence pledge or a virginity pledge. These are formal, written commitments or "contracts" saying that you promise to remain a virgin until marriage. Or, if you have had sex before, you promise to remain abstinent from that point until you get married. Abstinence pledges can be obtained through churches and Christian organizations such as True Love Waits and Silver Ring Thing. For some teens, it helps their resolve to have formally made a pledge to themselves and others.

You can also make a private pledge of abstinence to yourself or with a friend or group of friends. The wording and details of your pledge are up to you. A 2005 study from the Prevention Research Center in Berkeley, California, shows that teens are more likely to wait longer to begin having sex if they make an informal pledge to themselves or friends than if they sign a formal pledge associated with an organization.

No matter what level of abstinence you choose, it is still very important for you to be responsible for your own health and well-being. Take the time to learn about sexually transmitted diseases, how you can contract them, and where to find and how to use both condoms and other forms of contraception.

chapter three
Potential Consequences of Sexual Activity

One of the ways we figure out whether we have made a good decision is to look at the consequences (outcomes or effects) of the decision. Satisfactory long-term outcomes usually mean that a good decision was made. Undesirable outcomes, on the other hand, indicate that a poor decision was made. To make a good decision about your own sexual activity, you need to understand the health-related outcomes of failing to practice safer sex. These include sexually transmitted diseases (STDs) and

Before you become sexually active, both you and your partner should understand all the possible outcomes of having sex.

Potential Consequences of Sexual Activity

pregnancy. You also need to be aware of the difficult thoughts and emotions that can rise to the surface after you become sexually active.

Choosing to remain abstinent does not guarantee that you won't have to deal with any negative outcomes. Your friends, for example, may not initially respect your decision and might call you a "queer" or a "prude." These names can hurt, but they reflect your friends' ignorance more than anything else. What's important is that you understand your options and make the decision that you think is best for you at the time.

Sexually Transmitted Diseases (STDs)

It's a little scary to think about, but one wrong choice can result in a sexually transmitted disease. STDs can come from bacteria, parasites, microbes, or viruses. As you read earlier, these STDs are transmitted by blood, vaginal fluids, pre-ejaculatory fluid, and semen during sexual activity.

Some STDs produce very obvious symptoms, such as a burning sensation during urination or abnormal discharge from the vagina or penis. However, other STDs may have no symptoms at all and can be detected only through a doctor's tests. What you need to know is that, more often than not, someone with an STD shows few or no outward symptoms. This means there may be no obvious marks, sores, welts, or swelling to indicate that there is a problem. Affected people may look and generally feel completely normal. Because they feel just fine, they might think it is OK to have unprotected sex.

Making Smart Choices About Sexual Activity

Your partner might not tell you the truth if he or she has an STD. This could be because of feelings of embarrassment or shame, or the fear that you will want to break up if you know about it. So, even if you do trust your partner, it is in your own best interest to be careful. If your partner has been sexually active in any way before dating you, you should assume that there is a risk of contracting an STD from him or her.

STDs Caused by Bacteria

Chlamydia, gonorrhea, and syphilis are the three most common STDs caused by bacteria. Symptoms of both chlamydia and gonorrhea may include pain and burning while urinating and discharge from the penis or vagina. However, there may be no symptoms at all. Syphilis often causes sores on the anus, mouth, or genitals, but it may also have few or no symptoms. Syphilis may cause serious health issues and can even be fatal. All three of these bacterial STDs are treated with antibiotics, but strains of both gonorrhea and syphilis have become resistant to some antibiotics, making the STDs harder to treat.

STDs Caused by Parasites

Two common STDs caused by parasites are trichomoniasis and crab lice. These parasites can affect both guys and girls. Symptoms of trichomoniasis include itching or burning of the genital areas and pain while urinating. For women, symptoms may also include a yellow-green

Potential Consequences of Sexual Activity

vaginal discharge that is often accompanied by odor. Trichomoniasis can be treated with antibiotics.

Crab lice, or pubic lice, are generally found in pubic hair. Crab lice attach to the skin and hair and cause itching and irritation. Crab lice can be spread during sex when the pubic regions touch or from sharing the bedding of an infected person. (The lice can live in bedding for up to seven days.) Crab lice infestation is treated by shaving the pubic hair and washing the infected area with a special shampoo.

STDs Caused by Viruses

There are four STDs that are caused by viruses: HIV, HPV, hepatitis B, and herpes. It is the human immunodeficiency virus, or HIV, that will eventually cause the disease known as acquired immunodeficiency syndrome, or AIDS. HIV attacks the immune system and causes the body to be incapable of fighting

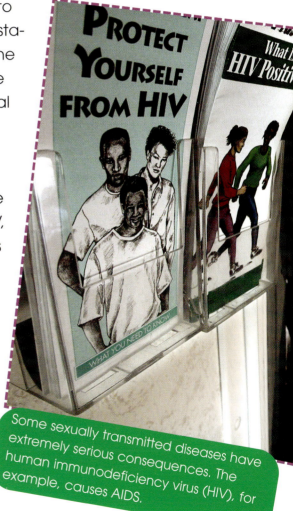

Some sexually transmitted diseases have extremely serious consequences. The human immunodeficiency virus (HIV), for example, causes AIDS.

off infections and diseases. The virus is contracted most commonly through sexual intercourse or by the sharing of needles. The only way to detect HIV is through a blood test. At present, AIDS is still considered to be a fatal disease. However, the early stages of HIV can be managed by a "cocktail" of various drugs that is generally successful in delaying the onset of AIDS.

The human papillomavirus, or HPV, generally causes small, white, cauliflower-like warts to appear on or around the genital area or inside the vagina or penis. Even if the warts are surgically removed by a doctor, the virus may still be spread through skin-to-skin contact and sexual intercourse. Some strains of HPV cause cervical cancer in women. A vaccine exists for the cancer-causing strains of HPV; you can discuss the pros and cons of taking this vaccine with your health-care provider.

Hepatitis B is the only STD that currently has a vaccine to prevent contracting the virus. Hepatitis B can be spread through the exchange of saliva, blood, semen, and vaginal fluid. The hepatitis B virus causes severe flu-like symptoms.

The herpes virus stays in your body for your entire life. Herpes can be treated to reduce symptoms, but it usually causes outbreaks of painful sores around the genital area, mouth, or anus.

Potential Outcome: Pregnancy

Reproduction is the natural purpose of sexual activity. So, obviously, one of the potential consequences of sexual

Potential Consequences of Sexual Activity

activity is pregnancy. Most teens, however, engage in sexual activity for a reason other than reproduction. The majority of teen pregnancies are not planned.

Recent government studies show that teen pregnancies in the United States are declining. In 2005, the birth rate was 21 per 1,000 women aged fifteen to seventeen. This marked an all-time low. (The rate for this group in 1991 was 39 births per 1,000 teenagers.)

How can a girl tell if she is pregnant? While each girl is different and the signs may vary, the most common signs of pregnancy are:

- A missed period
- Swollen and tender breasts
- Sleepiness
- Vomiting
- Frequent need to urinate

If you think you might be pregnant, you can buy a home pregnancy test from the drugstore or grocery store. These tests check your urine for an increase in certain hormone levels, which indicates pregnancy.

You can also visit your health-care provider or a family planning clinic such as Planned Parenthood. There, you can get a pregnancy test, and if you are pregnant, you can receive counseling and prenatal care for both you and your unborn baby. If you are pregnant, you have a choice to make. Among your options are:

Making Smart Choices About Sexual Activity

- Carrying your child to term and keeping the child
- Carrying the child to term and then putting the baby up for adoption
- Terminating the pregnancy (abortion)

Whichever option you choose, it is crucial that you discuss your options openly and honestly with both your healthcare provider and someone you trust. This could be one or both parents, a sibling or other family member, your school counselor, or your friends. Of course, you also need to talk frankly with the father of your unborn child. There are pros and cons associated with each of your options, and they need to be considered carefully. An unintended pregnancy is a very emotional and stressful time in a woman's life. It's good for a young woman to talk to those she loves and trusts to establish a support system for whatever decision she makes.

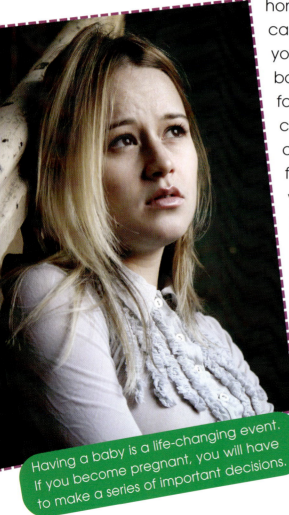

Having a baby is a life-changing event. If you become pregnant, you will have to make a series of important decisions.

Potential Consequences of Sexual Activity

Dealing with Emotions

Even the most confident teen may feel awkward around a boyfriend or girlfriend after having sex for the first time. Some may also feel confused or ashamed. Others may end up feeling alienated from their friends or family, especially if the teens' parents clearly disapprove of sex before marriage. These are all common feelings, but it's not healthy for you or your relationships to shut yourself away and worry. Instead, one of the best ways to help

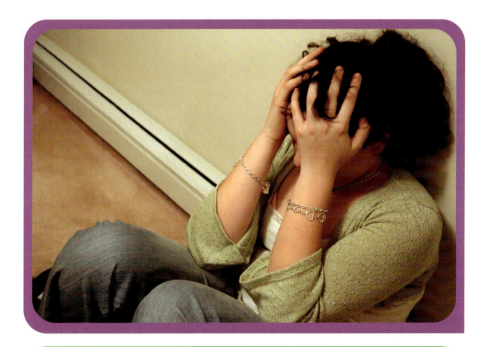

Having sex for the first time can unleash many strong emotions, including satisfaction and happiness. On the other hand, you may also feel shame, guilt, fear, anger, and sadness.

33

Making Smart Choices About Sexual Activity

yourself manage these feelings is to talk about them with someone you trust.

You may feel just as uncomfortable talking about the fact that you've had sex, but you'll find yourself feeling much better after getting your feelings off your chest. You might even find that the person you talk to has had the same feelings and can give you some good advice on how to handle the emotions you're experiencing.

Choosing Abstinence and Understanding the Emotions of Others

Some teens may use their sexuality as a way to cover up their lack of self-confidence. They'll decide to have sex in order to feel accepted or to get a certain guy or girl to like them. Or they believe that having sex will make them "cooler" and more grown-up. These people may be uncomfortable, even if they don't actually realize it, when one of their friends chooses to remain or become abstinent. Being abstinent can seem like a self-confident and independent choice, which may make someone who is not self-confident become more aware of his or her shortcomings.

If you have decided that you want to wait to have sex, you might find your friends giving you a hard time about your decision. They may try to make you feel that you are missing out on something or that you are somehow less cool. What you should realize is that your decision to be abstinent is probably not what is actually bothering them. Instead, your friends may be focusing on you because

Potential Consequences of Sexual Activity

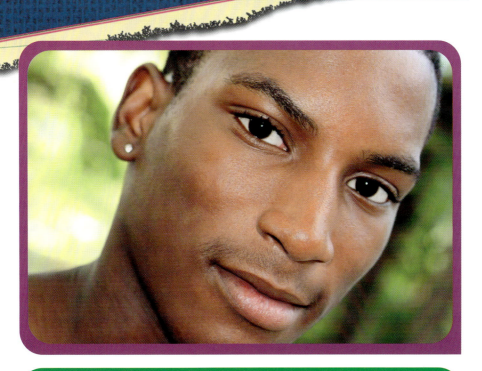

Waiting until you are emotionally ready to have sex is one of the best choices you can make. This decision shows that you know yourself and value your self-worth.

they are frustrated with their own lives and may be feeling shame or guilt about their own decision to have sex. Talk to them, be their friend, and continue being the same person you always have been with them. Eventually they will ease up on you, and down the road, they may even have great respect for your decision.

chapter four
Opportunities for Growth

This book was written to help you think your way through the big decision of whether or not to be sexually active. Such momentous decisions in our lives are never easy. When they come your way, it's best to be thoughtful and consider your options and all the possible outcomes. Sometimes, we try our best and still end up making a wrong choice. When this happens, it is important to remember that there is no such thing as being perfect. All of us occasionally make mistakes. But it is how we handle ourselves afterward that is a true measure

When you respect your partner and yourself, chances are good that you will make the right choices.

Opportunities for Growth

of who we are. Learning from your mistakes is how you grow into a better person.

Nobody Should Be Alone

While it is good to be independent, you don't have to face difficult choices alone. Should you find yourself dealing with an STD or unintended pregnancy, there is always someone you can get in touch with to discuss your options or to get assistance. You might feel most comfortable going to someone whom you know well, such as a parent, sibling, or friend. Or you might want to talk with someone

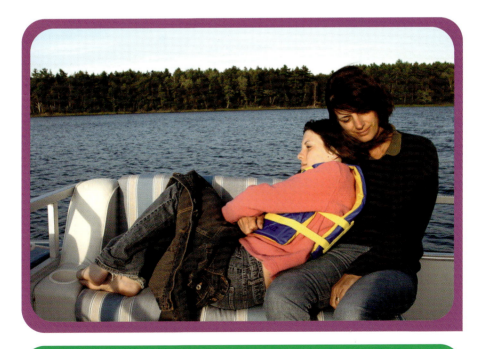

Confiding in someone you trust can make your burden less difficult. His or her past experiences may even help you to make better decisions in the future.

Making Smart Choices About Sexual Activity

who isn't so close to you, such as your health-care provider, your school counselor, or a counselor at a family planning clinic. You can even talk to a counselor anonymously via telephone hotlines.

Being at a crossroads can cause you to feel stress. During these times, sports and other types of exercise offer stress relief and other health benefits. You could also join youth groups that are available through your school or place of worship. Or you could just go buy a journal and write down your thoughts about all your choices and, eventually, the decision you make.

In Conclusion

You may decide that you want to remain abstinent for the time being, or until you meet that right person and get married. This is a choice that will probably be tough to live with at times. But in the end, sticking to your beliefs can bolster your self-confidence. On the other hand, you may feel that the time is right for you to begin having sex. If that's the case, you should be mature enough to communicate honestly with your partner. Talk about all aspects of having sex, both positive and negative. Doing this shows respect for both yourself and your partner. You can also show maturity and responsibility by going to a drugstore or family planning clinic to get latex condoms. To make an even smarter choice, always have safer sex by adding the contraceptive protection of spermicides and/or birth control pills.

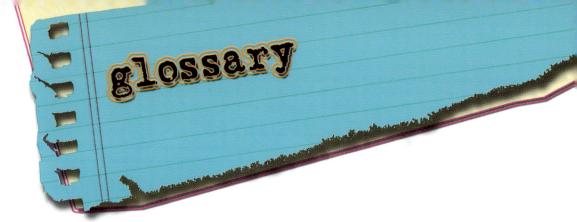

glossary

abstinence Practice of not having sex.

abstinence pledge/virginity pledge Formal or informal pledge to remain abstinent, usually until marriage.

acquired immunodeficiency syndrome (AIDS) Fatal disease caused by the human immunodeficiency virus (HIV).

birth control pills Hormone pills that prevent pregnancy in a female by stopping the ovulation process.

chlamydia Treatable sexually transmitted disease caused by bacteria.

condom Barrier method of contraception in the form of a latex sheath that fits over a man's penis.

contraception Prevention of pregnancy. Contraception includes condoms, birth control pills, and spermicides.

crab lice Tiny parasites that live in the pubic hair and in bedding; considered a sexually transmitted disease.

gonorrhea Bacterial infection that can cause major health problems if left untreated. Can have either no symptoms or a pain and burning while urinating.

hepatitis B Sexually transmitted disease that can be caused by the exchange of saliva. Causes serious flu-like symptoms.

Making Smart Choices About Sexual Activity

herpes Incurable sexually transmitted disease that causes painful sores on the mouth, anus, and genitals.

human immunodeficiency virus (HIV) Virus that attacks the immune system. It is transmitted during sex and through the sharing of needles.

human papillomavirus (HPV) Virus that often causes small, white, cauliflower-like warts on the genital area and inside the penis and vagina. Some strains of HPV can cause cervical cancer in women.

ovulation Process in a woman whereby one of her ovaries releases a mature egg that can then be fertilized by a man's sperm.

pre-ejaculatory fluid Bodily fluid that appears at the tip of the penis prior to ejaculation.

refrain To keep oneself from doing.

semen Sperm-containing fluid that comes from a man's penis when he ejaculates.

sexual activity Willing participation in sexual behaviors with another person.

sexual intercourse Act of penetration of a woman's vagina by a man's penis.

sexually transmitted disease (STD) A disease that can arise from sexual activity.

spermicide Chemicals that kill sperm.

trichomoniasis Common and curable sexually transmitted disease caused by a parasite that can cause painful urination and a yellow-green vaginal discharge.

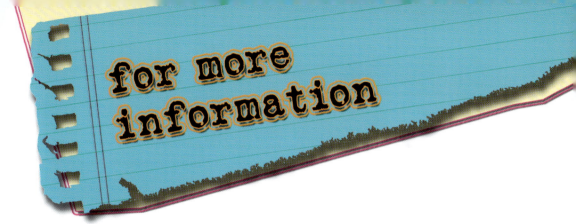

for more information

Abstinence Clearinghouse
801 East 41st Street
Sioux Falls, SD 57105
(605) 335-3643
Web site: http://www.abstinence.net
Abstinence Clearinghouse is a nonprofit organization supporting the abstinence community. It promotes the appreciation for and practice of sexual abstinence through distribution of age-appropriate, factual, and medically accurate materials.

Advocates for Youth
2000 M Street NW, Suite 750
Washington, DC 20036
(202) 419-3420
Web site: http://www.advocatesforyouth.org
Advocates for Youth is committed to advocating policies and creating informative programs that give young people the best information and resources for making educated decisions about their sexual and reproductive health.

Making Smart Choices About Sexual Activity

National Campaign to Prevent Teen Pregnancy
1776 Massachusetts Avenue NW, Suite 200
Washington, DC 20036
(202) 478-8500
Web site: http://www.teenpregnancy.org
The National Campaign to Prevent Teen Pregnancy is a nonprofit organization dedicated to reducing teen pregnancy and improving the well-being of children, youth, and families.

Planned Parenthood Federation of America
810 Seventh Avenue
New York, NY 10019
(800) 230-7526
Web site: http://www.plannedparenthood.org
Planned Parenthood has more than 860 affiliated health-care and family planning centers nationwide that offer health services regardless of age, income, race, or marital status. Planned Parenthood offers such services as STD testing and treatment, pregnancy testing, family planning, gynecological care, and birth control.

Web Sites

Due to the changing nature of Internet links, Rosen Publishing has developed an online list of Web sites related to the subject of this book. This site is updated regularly. Please use this link to access the list:

http://www.rosenlinks.com/msc/seac

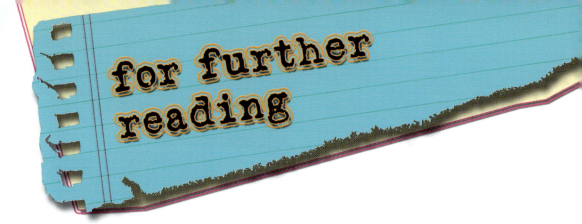

for further reading

Basso, Michael J. *The Underground Guide to Teenage Sexuality*. 2nd ed. New York, NY: Fairview Press, 2003.

Bell, Ruth. *Changing Bodies, Changing Lives: Expanded Third Edition: A Book for Teens on Sex and Relationships*. New York, NY: Three Rivers Press, 1998.

Connell, Elizabeth. *The Contraception Sourcebook*. New York, NY: McGraw-Hill, 2001.

Lange, Donna, and Mary Ann McDonnell. *Taking Responsibility: A Teen's Guide to Contraception and Pregnancy*. Broomall, PA: Mason Crest Publishers, 2004.

Lieberman, E. James, M.D., and Karen Lieberman Troccoli. *Like It Is: A Teen Sex Guide*. Jefferson, NC: McFarland, 1998.

Little, Marjorie. *Sexually Transmitted Diseases*. New York, NY: Chelsea House Publishers, 1999.

Pardes, Bronwen. *Doing It Right*. New York, NY: Simon & Schuster Children's, 2007.

Peacock, Judith. *Birth Control and Protection: Options for Teens*. Mankato, MN: LifeMatters, 2001.

Pogany, Susan. *Sex Smart: 501 Reasons to Hold Off on Sex*. New York, NY: Fairview Press, 1998.

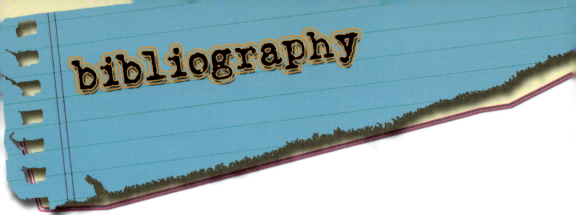

bibliography

Abma, J. C., G. M. Martinez, W. D. Mosner, and B. S. Dawson. "Teenagers in the United States: Sexual Activity, Contraceptive Use, and Childbearing, 2002." National Center for Health Statistics. *Vital Health Statistics*, Vol. 23, No. 24, 2004, pp. 1–48.

Advocates for Youth. "Adolescent Protective Behaviors: Abstinence and Contraceptive Use." Retrieved May 8, 2007 (http://www.advocatesforyouth.org/PUBLICATIONS/factsheet/fsprotective.htm).

Baumgardner, Jennifer. "Would You Pledge Your Virginity to Your Father?" Retrieved June 4, 2007 (http://www.glamour.com/news/articles/2007/01/purityballs07feb).

Bearman, P. S., and H. Brückner. *Promising the Future: Virginity Pledges as They Affect Transition to First Intercourse*. New York, NY: Columbia University, 2000.

Boodman, Sandra G. "Virginity Pledges Can't Be Taken on Faith." Retrieved June 4, 2007 (http://www.washingtonpost.com/wp-dyn/content/article/2006/05/15/AR2006051500842.html).

Brown, J. D., K. L. L'Engle, C. J. Pardun, G. Guo, K. Kenneavy, and C. Jackson. "Sexy Media Matter: Exposure to Sexual Content in Music, Movies, Television, and Magazines Predicts Black and White Adolescents'

Bibliography

Sexual Behavior." *Pediatrics*, Vol. 117, No. 4, April 2006, pp. 1,018–1,027.

Broyles, Matthew. "Abstinence." Teen Health and Wellness: Real Life, Real Answers. 2007. Rosen Publishing Group, Inc. Retrieved May 31, 2008 (http://www.thwrlra.com/article/26).

Brückner, H., and P. Bearman. "After the Promise: The STD Consequences of Adolescent Virginity Pledges." *Journal of Adolescent Health*, Vol. 36, No. 4, April 2005, pp. 271–278.

The Center for Young Women's Health. "Birth Control Pills." Retrieved June 12, 2007 (http://www.youngwomenshealth.org/femalehormone1.html).

Centers for Disease Control and Prevention. "Sexually Transmitted Diseases Fact Sheets." Retrieved June 2, 2007 (http://www.cdc.gov/std/healthcomm/fact_sheets.htm).

Centers for Disease Control and Prevention. "Sexually Transmitted Diseases Treatment Guidelines 2006." Retrieved June 2, 2007 (http://www.cdc.gov/STD/treatment/2006/toc.htm).

Centers for Disease Control and Prevention. "Trends in Reportable Sexually Transmitted Diseases in the United States, 2003—National Data on Chlamydia, Gonorrhea and Syphilis." Retrieved June 2, 2007 (http://www.cdc.gov/std/stats03/trends2003.htm).

Connolly, Ceci. "Some Abstinence Programs Mislead Teens, Report Says." Retrieved June 4, 2007 (http://www.washingtonpost.com/wp-dyn/articles/A26623-2004Dec1.html).

Greenberger, Robert. "Safe Sex." Teen Health and Wellness: Real Life, Real Answers. 2007. Rosen Publishing Group, Inc. Retrieved June 4, 2007 (http://www.thwrlra.com/article/287).

Knowles, Jon, Jennifer Johnsen, and Chelsea Nelson. "Guide for Teens & Families." Retrieved May 8, 2007 (http://www.plannedparenthood.org/sexual-health/teens-health/guide-for-teens-and-families.htm).

The National Campaign to Prevent Teen Pregnancy. "National Teen Pregnancy and Birth Data General Facts and Stats." Retrieved May 2, 2007 (http://www.teenpregnancy.org/resources/data/genlfact.asp).

Science Daily. "U.S. Teen Pregnancy Rates Decline as Result of Improved Contraceptive Use." Retrieved June 4, 2007 (http://www.sciencedaily.com/releases/2006/12/061201180530.htm).

U.S. Department of Health and Human Services' WomensHealth.gov. "Birth Control Methods." Retrieved June 12, 2007 (http://www.womenshealth.gov/faq/birthcont.htm).

Weiss, Deborah. "Pregnancy and Childbearing Among U.S. Teens." Retrieved May 2, 2007 (http://www.plannedparenthood.org/news-articles-press/politics-policy-issues/teen-pregnancy-sex-education/teen-pregnancy-6239.htm).

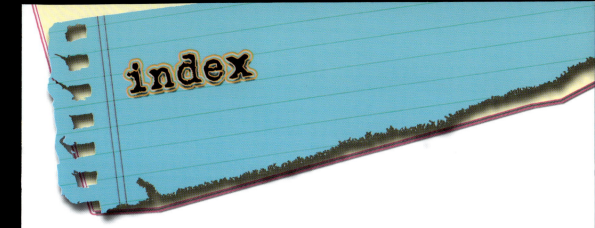

index

A
abstinence, 10–11, 17, 23–25, 27, 34, 38
Abstinence Clearinghouse, 25
abstinence/virginity pledge, 25
abstinence support groups, 25
AIDS, 29, 30

B
birth control pills, 20, 21, 38

C
cervical cancer, 30
chlamydia, 28
condoms, 17, 20–21, 22, 25, 38
contraception, 20–22, 25, 38
crab lice, 28–29

G
gonorrhea, 28

H
hepatitis B, 29, 30
herpes, 18, 29, 30
HIV, 18, 29–30
HPV, 29, 30

M
media, 8–9
mistakes, making, 5–6, 36–37

O
ovulation, 21, 22

P
Planned Parenthood, 31
pregnancy, 5, 11, 13, 15, 18–19, 20, 21, 22, 27, 30–32, 37
pregnancy tests, 31
pressure, 11, 13, 14, 23

R
role models, 7–8

S
safe sex, 5, 17, 19–20, 26, 38
self-confidence/self-esteem, 5, 23, 33, 34, 38
self-image/identity, 5, 7
sexual activity, explanation of, 9–10
sexually transmitted diseases (STDs), 5, 11, 12, 13, 18, 20, 22, 23, 25, 26, 27, 28, 37

transmission of, 12–13, 20–21, 27, 29, 30
    types of, 28–30
Silver Ring Thing, 25
spermicides, 20, 22, 38

syphilis, 28

T

trichomoniasis, 28–29
True Love Waits, 25

About the Author

Stephanie C. Perkins is a writer and editor who lives and works in Houston, Texas. Although her writing has taken her in many directions over the years, she always gravitates back to health-related topics and feels a great responsibility to educate young people about their health and how best to take care of themselves. Perkins has written extensively for Rosen's Teen Health and Wellness database. In her spare time, she is hard at work on her first novel.

Photo Credits

Cover © www.istockphoto.com/Shelly Perry; p. 4 © www.istockphoto.com/TriggerPhoto; p. 7 © Bob Daemmrich/The Image Works; p. 10 © www.istockphoto.com/Liz Van Steenburgh; p. 12 © Michael Newman/PhotoEdit; p. 14 © www.istockphoto.com/Wendy Nero; p. 16 © www.istockphoto.com/Justin Horrocks; p. 18 © www.istockphoto.com/Izabela Habur; p. 21 © William B. Plowman/Getty Images; p. 24 © www.istockphoto.com/Chris Schmidt; p. 26 © John Berry/Syracuse Newspapers/The Image Works; p. 29 © Spencer Platt/Getty Images; p. 32 © www.istockphoto.com/Stockphoto4u; p. 33 © www.istockphoto.com/Jim Lopes; p. 35 © www.istockphoto.com/Eileen Hart; p. 36 © www.istockphoto.com/Viktor Pryymachuk; p. 37 © James Marshall/The Image Works.

Designer: Tahara Anderson; **Editor**: Christopher Roberts
Photo Researcher: Amy Feinberg

Date Due

BRODART, CO.   Cat. No. 23-233   Printed in U.S.A.